INDIGESTION CURE

An essential guide on how to take care of indigestion

Dr Rowan Theo

Table of Contents

CHAPTER ONE

INDIGESTION CURE

How to Treat Indigestion at Home

Your favored meals can satisfaction your flavor buds. But in case you consume too rapid or eat an excessive amount of those meals, you can enjoy occasional indigestion.

Symptoms of indigestion can consist of uncomfortable belly fullness after ingesting, or you can have ache or a burning sensation for your top belly.

Indigestion isn't a disease, however as an alternative a symptom of different gastrointestinal issues, inclusive of an ulcer, gastritis, or acid reflux disease disorder.

Many humans may have indigestion at a few point. Instead of achieving for over the counter antacids to calm your belly, you would possibly need to attempt controlling signs and symptoms with components and herbs for your kitchen.

Here's a have a take a observe 8 domestic treatments that may offer short comfort for indigestion.

Peppermint tea

Peppermint is greater than a breath freshener. It additionally has an antispasmodic impact at the frame, making it a excellent desire for alleviating belly issues like nausea and indigestion. Drink a cup of peppermint tea after food to speedy soothe your belly or maintain some portions of peppermint for your pocket and suck at the sweet after ingesting.

While peppermint can ease indigestion, you shouldn't drink or consume peppermint whilst indigestion is resulting from acid reflux disease disorder. Because peppermint relaxes the decrease esophageal sphincter — the muscle among the belly and the esophagus — ingesting or ingesting it is able to reason belly acid to go with the drift again into the esophagus and get worse acid reflux disease disorder. Peppermint tea isn't always advocated for humans with GERD or ulcers.

Chamomile tea

Chamomile tea is thought to assist set off sleep and calm anxiety. This herb also can ease intestine soreness and relieve indigestion via way of means of decreasing belly acid in the gastrointestinal tract. Chamomile additionally acts as an anti inflammatory to prevent ache.

To put together chamomile tea, region one or teabags in boiling water for 10 mins. Pour in a cup and upload honey, if desired. Drink the tea as had to prevent indigestion.

Consult a physician earlier than ingesting chamomile tea in case you take a blood thinner. Chamomile consists of an element that acts as an anticoagulant, so there's the danger of bleeding whilst blended with a blood thinner.

Apple cider vinegar

The claimed fitness advantages of apple cider vinegar variety from enhancing the situation of pores and skin to encouraging weight loss. It may assist to ease indigestion.

Since too little belly acid can cause indigestion, drink apple cider vinegar to boom your frame's manufacturing of belly acid. Add one to 2 teaspoons of uncooked, unpasteurized apple cider vinegar to a cup of water and drink for immediate comfort. Or prevent indigestion earlier than it takes place via way of means of ingesting the combination half-hour earlier than ingesting.

Even aleven though apple cider vinegar is secure, ingesting it in extra or undiluted can reason facet consequences inclusive of teeth erosion, nausea, throat burn, and coffee blood sugar.

Ginger

Ginger is any other herbal treatment for indigestion due to the fact it is able to lessen belly acid. The equal manner too little belly acid reasons indigestion, an excessive amount of belly acid has the equal impact.

Drink a cup of ginger tea as had to soothe your belly and take away indigestion. Other alternatives consist of sucking on ginger sweet, ingesting ginger ale, or making your very own ginger water. Boil one or portions of ginger root in 4 cups of water. Add taste with lemon or honey earlier than ingesting.

Limit your ginger intake to . Consuming an excessive amount of ginger can reason fueloline, throat burn, and heartburn.

Fennel seed

This antispasmodic herb also can treatment indigestion after a meal, in addition to soothe different gastrointestinal issues like belly cramping, nausea, and bloating.

Put half of teaspoon of beaten fennel seed in water and permit it to boil for 10 mins earlier than ingesting. Drink fennel tea each time you enjoy indigestion. Another choice is to bite fennel seed after food if positive meals reason indigestion.

Possible facet consequences of fennel consist of nausea, vomiting, and solar sensitivity.

CHAPTER TWO

Baking soda (sodium bicarbonate)

Baking soda can speedy neutralize belly acid and relieve indigestion, bloating, and fueloline after ingesting. For this treatment, upload half of teaspoon of baking soda to four oz. of heat water and drink.

Sodium bicarbonate is typically secure and nontoxic. But ingesting huge quantities of baking soda can bring about some unwelcome facet consequences, inclusive of constipation, diarrhea, irritability, vomiting, and muscle spasms. If you drink an answer containing half of teaspoon of baking soda for indigestion, don't repeat for at the least hours.

adults have to haven't any greater than seven half of teaspoons in a 24-hour length and no greater than 3 half of teaspoons if over the age of 60.

7. Lemon water

The alkaline impact of lemon water additionally neutralizes belly acid and improves digestion. Mix a tablespoon of lemon juice in warm or heat water and drink a couple of minutes earlier than ingesting.

Along with easing indigestion, lemon water is additionally an exquisite supply of diet C. However, an excessive amount of lemon water can put on down teeth and reason accelerated urination. To defend your teeth, rinse your mouth with water after ingesting lemon water.

8. Licorice root

Licorice root can calm muscle spasms and infection in the gastrointestinal tract, which each can cause indigestion. Chew licorice root for comfort or upload licorice root to boiling water and drink the combination.

Although powerful for indigestion, licorice root can reason sodium and potassium imbalances and excessive blood strain in huge doses. Consume no greater than 2.five grams of dried licorice root consistent with day for immediate comfort. Eat or drink licorice root half-hour earlier than ingesting or one hour after ingesting for indigestion.

Buy licorice root.

When to peer a physician

Even aleven though indigestion is a common hassle, a few bouts shouldn't be ignored. Frequent indigestion is usually a symptom of a continual digestive hassle like acid reflux disease disorder, gastritis, or even belly cancer. Therefore, see a physician if indigestion maintains for greater than weeks, or in case you enjoy intense ache or different signs and symptoms inclusive of:

• weight loss

• lack of appetite

• vomiting

• black stools

• hassle swallowing

• fatigue

The takeaway

You don't must stay with common indigestion. Stomach soreness can disrupt your life, however it doesn't must. See if those domestic treatments assist however go to a physician approximately any worrisome signs and symptoms.

The FDA doesn't display herbs and treatments for great, so studies your emblem choices.

The quicker you spot a physician, get a diagnosis, and start remedy, the earlier you could experience higher and revel in a better great of life.

Ways to Prevent Heartburn and Acid Reflux

Most people are all too acquainted with the painful, burning sensation in the middle of the chest that's related to heartburn.

In fact, as much as 28% of adults in North America enjoy gastroesophageal reflux disease (GERD), a common situation that reasons heartburn. GERD takes place whilst acid is driven up from the belly again into the esophagus, which results in the heartburn sensation (1).

Although humans frequently use medicinal drugs to deal with acid reflux disease disorder and heartburn, many life-style adjustments also can assist you lessen signs and symptoms and enhance your great of life.

CHAPTER THREE

Home Remedies for Heartburn and Acid Reflux

1. Chew gum

A few older research have proven that chewing gum might also additionally assist lower acidity in the esophagus (2, 3, 4).

Gum that consists of bicarbonate seems to be specially powerful, as it is able to assist neutralize acid to save you reflux.

Chewing gum also can boom saliva manufacturing, which might also additionally assist clean the esophagus of acid.

However, greater up to date studies is wanted to decide whether or not chewing gum can assist deal with acid reflux disease disorder or relieve the signs and symptoms of heartburn.

SUMMARY

Chewing gum will increase the formation of saliva and might assist clean the esophagus of belly acid.

2. Sleep for your left facet

Several research have determined that slumbering for your proper facet might also additionally get worse reflux signs and symptoms at night time .

In fact, in keeping with one evaluate, mendacity for your left facet might also additionally lower acid publicity in the esophagus via way of means of as much as 71%.

Although the motive isn't always completely clean, it is able to be defined via way of means of anatomy.

The esophagus enters the proper facet of the belly. As a result, the decrease esophageal sphincter sits above the extent of belly acid while you sleep for your left facet.

On the opposite hand, while you lie for your proper facet, belly acid covers the decrease esophageal sphincter, growing the danger of reflux .

While slumbering at the left facet all night time won't continually be possible, it is able to assist make you greater snug as you fall asleep.

SUMMARY

If you enjoy acid reflux disease disorder at night time, attempt slumbering at the left facet of your frame.

3 Elevate the pinnacle of your mattress

Some humans enjoy reflux signs and symptoms at some point of the night time, that can have an effect on sleep great and make it greater tough to fall asleep .

Changing the placement which you sleep in via way of means of raising the pinnacle of your mattress may want to assist lessen signs and symptoms of acid reflux disease disorder and enhance sleep great.

One evaluate of 4 research determined that raising the pinnacle of the mattress reduced acid reflux disease disorder and stepped forward signs and symptoms like heartburn and regurgitation in humans with

Another examine confirmed that those who used a wedge to raise their top frame whilst slumbering skilled much less acid reflux disease disorder as compared with after they slept flat .

SUMMARY

Elevating the pinnacle of your mattress might also additionally lessen your reflux signs and symptoms at night time.

4. Eat dinner in advance

Healthcare specialists frequently endorse humans with acid reflux disease disorder to keep away from ingesting in the three hours earlier than they visit sleep.

That's due to the fact mendacity horizontally after a meal makes digestion greater tough, doubtlessly worsening GERD signs and symptoms.

According to at least one evaluate, ingesting a past due-dinner party accelerated acid publicity whilst mendacity down via way of means of five%, as compared with ingesting in advance in the nighttime.

SUMMARY

Observational research advocate that ingesting near bedtime might also additionally get worse acid reflux disease disorder signs and symptoms at night time. However, the proof is inconclusive, and greater research are wished.

5 Opt for cooked onions in preference to uncooked

Raw onions are a commoncause for acid reflux disease disorder and heartburn.

One older examine in humans with acid reflux disease disorder confirmed that ingesting a meal containing uncooked onion drastically accelerated heartburn, acid reflux disease disorder, and burping, as compared with eating an equal meal that didn't comprise onions.

More common burping would possibly advocate that greater fueloline is being produced. This will be because of the excessive quantities of fermentable fiber in onions.

Raw onions also are greater tough to digest and may worsen the liner of the esophagus, inflicting worsened heartburn.

Whatever the motive, in case you suppose ingesting uncooked onion makes your signs and symptoms worse, you have to keep away from it and choose cooked onions instead.

SUMMARY

Some humans enjoy worsened heartburn and different reflux signs and symptoms after ingesting uncooked onions.

CHAPTER FOUR

Eat smaller, greater common food

There's a ring-like muscle called the decrease esophageal sphincter wherein the esophagus opens into the belly.

It acts as a valve and typically prevents the acidic contents of the belly from going up into the esophagus. It commonly remains closed however might also additionally open while you swallow, belch, or vomit.

In humans with acid reflux disease disorder, this muscle is weakened or dysfunctional. Acid reflux also can arise whilst there's an excessive amount of strain at the muscle, inflicting acid to squeeze via the opening.

Unsurprisingly, maximum reflux signs and symptoms take region after a meal. It additionally appears that ingesting simply one to 2 huge food consistent with day might also additionally get worse reflux signs and symptoms.

Therefore, ingesting smaller, greater common food during the day might also additionally assist lessen signs and symptoms of acid reflux disease disorder.

SUMMARY

Acid reflux generally will increase after food, and large food appear to make it worse. Therefore, ingesting smaller, greater common food can be beneficial.

7. Maintain a slight weight

The diaphragm is a muscle placed above your belly. Normally, the diaphragm certainly strengthens the decrease esophageal sphincter, which prevents immoderate quantities of belly acid from leaking up into the esophagus.

However, when you have extra stomach fats, the strain for your stomach might also additionally come to be so excessive that the decrease esophageal sphincter receives driven upward, far from the diaphragm's support.

Achieving and retaining a slight frame weight can assist lessen acid reflux disease disorder in the lengthy term.

However, in case you're interested by this approach, make certain to talk with a healthcare expert to evaluate whether or not it's proper for you, and if so, how you could shed pounds accurately and sustainably.

SUMMARY

Losing stomach fats and retaining a slight weight would possibly relieve a number of your signs and symptoms of GERD. However, make certain to talk with a healthcare expert earlier than trying to shed pounds to deal with this situation.

8. Follow a low carb food plan

Growing proof shows that low carb diets might also additionally relieve acid reflux disease disorder signs and symptoms.

In fact, a few researchers suspect that undigested carbs might also additionally reason bacterial overgrowth and accelerated strain within the stomach, that can make contributions to acid reflux disease disorder.

Having too many undigested carbs for your digestive device frequently cannot simplest reason fueloline and bloating however additionally burping.

However, whilst a few research advocate that low carb diets may want to enhance reflux signs and symptoms, greater studies is wanted.

SUMMARY

Some studies shows that terrible carb digestion and bacterial overgrowth in the small gut might also additionally bring about acid reflux disease disorder. Low carb diets can be an powerful remedy, however in addition research are wished.

9. Limit your alcohol consumption

Drinking alcohol might also additionally boom the severity of acid reflux disease disorder and heartburn.

In fact, a few research have proven that better alcohol consumption will be related to accelerated signs and symptoms of acid reflux disease disorder.

Alcohol aggravates signs and symptoms via way of means of

growing belly acid, enjoyable the decrease esophageal sphincter, and impairing the cappotential of the esophagus to clean out acid.

Although new studies is wanted, a few older research additionally display that ingesting wine or beer will increase reflux signs and symptoms, specially as compared with ingesting undeniable water.

SUMMARY

Excessive alcohol consumption can get worse acid reflux disease disorder signs and symptoms. If you enjoy heartburn, proscribing your alcohol consumption would possibly assist ease a number of your soreness.

CHAPTER FIVE

Don't drink an excessive amount of espresso

Studies have determined that espresso briefly relaxes the decrease esophageal sphincter, growing the danger of acid reflux disease disorder.

Some proof additionally factors in the direction of caffeine as a likely reason. Similarly to espresso, caffeine relaxes the decrease esophageal sphincter, that can reason reflux.

Nevertheless, even though numerous research advocate that espresso and caffeine might also additionally get worse acid reflux disease disorder for a few humans, the proof isn't always completely conclusive.

For example, one evaluation of observational research determined no enormous consequences of espresso consumption at the self-said signs and symptoms of GERD.

Yet, whilst researchers investigated the symptoms and symptoms of acid reflux disease disorder with a small camera, they determined espresso intake changed into related to more acid harm in the esophagus .

Thus, whether or not espresso consumption worsens acid reflux disease disorder might also additionally rely on the individual. If you locate espresso offers you heartburn, it's great to actually keep away from it or restrict your consumption.

SUMMARY

Evidence shows that espresso might also additionally make acid reflux disease disorder and heartburn worse. If you experience like espresso worsens your signs and symptoms, keep in mind proscribing your consumption.

11. Limit your consumption of carbonated liquids

Healthcare specialists from time to time endorse humans with GERD to restrict their consumption of carbonated liquids.

This is due to the fact research have found that everyday intake of carbonated or fizzy liquids, inclusive of smooth drinks, membership soda, and seltzer, will be related to a better danger of reflux.

One examine determined that carbonated smooth drinks, in particular, worsened positive acid reflux disease disorder signs and symptoms, inclusive of heartburn, fullness, and burping.

The principal motive is that the carbon dioxide fueloline (the bubbles) in carbonated liquids reasons humans to burp greater frequently — an impact that may boom the quantity of acid escaping into the esophagus.

SUMMARY

Drinking carbonated liquids briefly will increase the frequency of burping, which might also additionally sell acid reflux disease disorder. If they get worse your signs and symptoms, attempt ingesting much less or warding off them altogether.

12. Don't drink an excessive amount of citrus juice

Many forms of citrus juice, inclusive of orange juice and grapefruit juice, are taken into consideration common triggers for heartburn.

These components are quite acidic and comprise compounds like ascorbic acid, that can reason indigestion in case you eat them in huge quantities.

In addition to being acidic, positive compounds determined in citrus juice may want to worsen the liner of the esophagus.

While citrus juice possibly doesn't reason acid reflux disease disorder directly, it is able to make your heartburn worse briefly.

SUMMARY

Some humans with acid reflux disease disorder file that ingesting citrus juice makes their signs and symptoms worse. Certain compounds in citrus juice, similarly to acids, also can worsen the liner of the esophagus.

13. Avoid mint, if wished

Peppermint and spearmint are common components used to make natural tea and upload taste to meals, sweet, chewing gum, mouthwash, and toothpaste.

However, additionally they comprise positive compounds that might cause heartburn in a few humans.

For instance, a few research suggest that peppermint oil may want to lower decrease esophageal sphincter strain, which might also additionally reason heartburn.

Another examine confirmed that menthol, a compound determined in mint, may want to get worse reflux in humans with GERD.

Additionally, one older examine in humans with GERD confirmed that spearmint did now no longer have an effect on the decrease esophageal sphincter. Nevertheless, it determined that excessive doses of spearmint may want to get worse acid reflux disease disorder signs and symptoms via way of means of annoying the inner of the esophagus.

For this motive, it's great to keep away from mint in case you experience that it makes your heartburn worse.

SUMMARY

A few research suggest that mint and a number of the compounds it consists of might also additionally worsen heartburn and different reflux signs and symptoms, however the proof is limited.

CHAPTER SIX

Limit excessive fats meals

Fried meals and a few different fatty meals can also be a cause for GERD. Some studies indicates they will result in heartburn. Examples consist of.

- fried meals

- potato chips

- pizza

- bacon

- sausage

High fats meals like those might also additionally make contributions to heartburn via way of means of inflicting bile salts to be launched into your digestive tract, which might also additionally worsen your esophagus.

They additionally seem to stimulate the discharge of cholecystokinin (CCK), a hormone for your bloodstream which could loosen up the decrease esophageal sphincter, permitting belly contents again into the esophagus.

One examine checked out what befell whilst humans with GERD ate excessive fats meals. More than 1\/2 of contributors who had said meals triggers stated they skilled GERD signs and symptoms after ingesting excessive fats, fried meals.

Moreover, as soon as those humans removed triggering meals from their food plan, the percentage of individuals who skilled heartburn reduced from 93% to 44%.

More studies is wanted to discover how excessive fats meals would possibly cause GERD signs and symptoms, inclusive of heartburn, in addition to what types of fat would possibly have the most powerful consequences.

It's crucial to be aware that fat are an important a part of a healthful food plan. Rather than warding off fat, purpose to consume them carefully from healthful sources, inclusive of omega-three fatty acids from fatty fish and monounsaturated fat from olive oil or avocados.

SUMMARY

Foods which can be excessive in fats might also additionally cause GERD signs and symptoms, inclusive of heartburn, in a few humans. However, greater studies is wanted.

The backside line

Heartburn is an uncomfortable difficulty that may be resulting from quite a few extraordinary factors.

Although there are numerous medicinal drugs and remedy alternatives to be had to ease heartburn, making some easy adjustments on your food plan and life-style can also be beneficial.

Try a number of the pointers above to locate what works so one can lessen heartburn and acid reflux disease disorder.

THE END